Dear God, I'm in Pain

28-Day Devotional For Those Who Are Suffering

BEEDA L. SPEIS

DEAR GOD LTD

This devotional is a work of original content and includes Bible verses from various translations. Scripture quotations marked (ESV) are from the ESV Bible (The Holy Bible, English Standard Version ®, copyright © 2001 by Crossway, a publishing ministry of Good News Publishers, Used by permission. All rights reserved.

Scripture quotations marked (NKJV) are from The Holy Bible, New Kings James Version, Copyright © 1979, 1980, 1982 by Thomas Nelson, Inc. Used by permission. All rights reserved.

E-book, devotional ASIN: B0CNX5CLJ3
Paperback devotional ISBN: 979-8-9896966-0-4

Audio-book, Narrated by Angela Ohlfest
https://www.fiverr.com/voiceoverangela
Cover design by Tayyab M @ Fiverr
https://www.fiverr.com/s/LkwXy4
Paperback journal ISBN: 979-8-9896966-1-1
Paperback pain tracker ISBN: 979-8-9896966-2-8

Dedication

This is for everyone suffering from chronic pain. Our families and friends can't fully understand us. Our physicians won't give us pain medication, so our only option is to suffer through the bad days and do what we can on our good ones.

However, we have access to The Great Physician. He hears our cries. He knows our pain. We may never know the reason for our suffering, but we can have a peace in knowing that everything happens for a reason (Romans 8:28).

Nothing is impossible for our God.

Acknowledgments

My deepest, most sincere gratitude to my family and friends who've supported my writing over the last ten + years. Without you, I would have given up long ago. It's your love and encouragement that led me to this very moment.

Table of Contents

prayer based on a topic for that week. Monday through Friday, I post about the topic, my life, anecdotes, songs, and/or images, etc., with a Bible verse and a prayer. Saturday and Sunday, I post an image with a verse on it. I called the group *7th Hour Prayer Power*. Later, the name was changed to *Pray in the Stillness* to align with my new branding and website, *Peace in the Stillness*. The idea behind it is that when we slow down and connect with God, we can find peace, *His* peace. All the trouble and pain of this world melt away when we're in His divine presence.

My first post, 9/23/2018:
The Power of Prayer
I've been in constant prayer for the last two weeks about all the spiritual and physical needs of the people in my life. I have felt so helpless and needed guidance. I wanted to be able to DO something, anything, to ease the burden on their hearts and to take away the pain and suffering. This morning, God blessed me with a task. I hope and pray that this will grow into an international daily event that will glorify God and show the world the power of prayer.

Tomorrow, during the 7 a.m. hour, set aside one minute to pray with me. It can be in your car on the way to work, in the shower, when you wake up, or sometime during that hour. Set an alarm, or write yourself a note. We will pray together on one particular people group a week.

I drew from those posts to develop this devotional. I chose the weeks we prayed for those who needed healing, those who had suffered, and a week when we prayed for peace for those who were sick or injured. I also took from the weeks we prayed about our hope in Jesus and our trust in the Lord.

Healing - this was a time of renewed confidence in the power of prayer for me. I just returned from a missions conference (the same conference I mentioned before, but two years earlier). We need to keep the faith. We need to pray for our own healing and ask others to pray for us, too. There's no shame in needing prayer. The ability to ask God for help is a blessing.

Suffering - Why must I suffer? I'm not trying to minimize anyone's pain by saying God has a purpose for it, for us. I know that's not necessarily helpful when you're in constant pain. It's difficult to understand why my pain is necessary. However, I feel like if I'm suffering for the glory of God, especially after everything Jesus endured to pay the price for my sins, then it's easier to handle and keeps me from despair. Despair is the work of Satan. He likes to put a wedge between us and our Creator.

Peace - It's challenging to have peace when we're in pain. We can't sleep, can't get comfortable. Some of us have relatives, loved ones, co-workers, and/or bosses who don't believe it's as bad as we claim. Most mornings, it's hard to even get out of bed. However, as Christians, we can find peace in our Savior.

Hope - Often, we hope things are different than they are. We pray a cure is found for our condition. We dream someone invents a magic pill that will take away all of our pain and not leave us feeling like zombies. The only true hope we have is what Jesus offers us. Cling to that hope. Find rest in it.

WEEK 1
HEALING

And the prayer of faith will save the sick, and the Lord will raise him up

James 5:15a

Let's Move Mountains

For assuredly, I say to you, whoever says to this mountain,
'Be removed and be cast into the sea,' and does not doubt in
his heart,
but believes that those things he says will be done,
he will have whatever he says.
Therefore I say to you,
whatever things you ask when you pray,
believe that you receive them,
and you will have them.
Mark 11:23-24 NKJV

This week, we're going to move mountains!

I just returned from a week of missions training, and my heart is renewed and strengthened for the power of prayer. I'm overflowing with the Holy Spirit, and I want to use this to help others. This week, let's pray BOLDLY! Believe in your heart that God can and will heal us. May God be glorified in the healing of His children.

The above paragraph is from a post I wrote in January 2020. My Facebook Group, *Pray in the Stillness*, and my blog followers, *Peace in the Stillness*, prayed for a list of people with various illnesses; some were life-threatening. They were all showing improvement, and then Covid hit. Four of them passed away, two of them I lost touch with, one is still surviving and living life to the fullest, and the last one, a little girl, has been completely healed.

The Bible tells us many times that if we have faith, if we *truly* believe, then God will grant us anything we pray for. We should be able to move that mountain with our sheer belief in the power of God. Yet, some of the things we pray for we don't receive. Why is that?

I always say that God answers every single one of my prayers. However, it may not be the answer I'm looking for and may not be in the time-frame I want. He is sovereign over all things, and I know that if I'm to continue in pain and fatigue, there must be a reason for it. He wants us to take everything to Him in prayer. It's one of the ways we get to know Him better. I repeat prayers daily until I receive an answer, and I understand that sometimes the answer is "no."

Dear GOD: I wish to move this mountain and cast it into the sea! My faith is strong. I believe in You, and I believe in Your word. If it be Your will, please take this pain from me. It is a mountain that blocks my path. I need You, dear Lord. In Jesus' name, I pray. Amen.

Prayer of Faith

And the prayer of faith will save the sick,
and the Lord will raise him up.
James 5:15a NKJV

I am fired up, having just spent a week among believers and those with a heart for mission work. I hope this energy for prayer and sharing never dies down, and you can feel it, too. Beginning with the first of the year, I started a prayer journal to remember everyone I'd promised to pray for. Also, it's a visual way to see God's response to our prayers.

Hopefully, you're familiar with George Muller. He was a Pastor in England who built and maintained several orphanages beginning in 1836. He never asked anyone for money to support the orphanages, but he prayed daily that God would supply all of their needs. His prayers were always answered. People would show up at his door and say something to the effect, "The Lord moved me to donate this money." It wasn't always money. People provided food, supplies, and services, but none were asked to do so. It was all God, and it was all in answer to prayers.

George Mueller also prayed continually for the unsaved by name. At the time of his death, only one person he knew of did not come to faith, but rumor has it that the man was saved after Mueller's death in 1898.

The power of prayer.

Dear GOD: may my prayer of faith save the sick, including my own issues and pain. I pray that You will raise me up. Heal me, Lord. I put my faith in You alone. In Jesus' name, I pray. Amen.

Confidence In Prayer

Now this is the confidence that we have in Him,
that if we ask anything according to His will,
He hears us.
1 John 5:14 NKJV

The home screen on my phone says: "Pray about everything. Philippians 4:6." I often look at my phone, so it is the perfect place to put such an important reminder.

These past three days of Bible verses have all had something in common. They all indicate that God will grant us whatever we ask for, if we have faith. Several of the verses this week say that, yet I'm confident that you, like me, have prayed exhaustively to be healed and for God to heal our friends. Yet, here we are. What should we make of that?

There are several answers that we need to **ignore**:

- Your faith isn't strong enough.
- God is punishing you.
- It's God's will.

I've read several commentaries on this and similar passages, and none of them explain it well enough for me to understand. What I *do* know is that the above three responses sound amazingly similar to the reasoning arguments of Job's "friends."

Maybe, like Job, you or I will get to the breaking point and cry out against our Maker, "Why?! Why are You doing this to me?" (Loosely paraphrased). And He may then ask us the questions He asked Job (Job 38-41).

Also, know that:

- No one knows how strong your faith is except you and God. Don't let others make you question it.

- God is not punishing you. We live in a fallen, sinful world in which bad things happen to good people. Jesus already took the punishment for our sins. Whatever you repent of is forgiven.

- It's not God's will that anyone should perish (2 Peter 3:9). This verse is for salvation, but I find it encouraging in other circumstances. Our God is a patient and loving Father. God most likely will use your pain; it may be part of the big picture, but it's not God's will that you should suffer.

Keep praying and believing. God hears you. Know that. Rest in it. He will never leave you nor forsake you (Deuteronomy 31:6b).

Dear God: I have confidence in You alone. I ask that, if it is Your will, please take this pain from me. I will wait on You, Lord. I will guard my heart with Your Spirit and not let others lead me astray. Only You know the reason for my pain, and I know that, in Your perfect timing, You will use this experience for Your glory. In Jesus' name, I pray. Amen.

Encouragement for the New Year

He will wipe every tear from their eyes. There will be
no more death or mourning or crying or pain, for the
old order of things has passed away.
Revelation 21:4 ESV

I've wanted to say something to you to comfort or inspire you,
but the words just haven't been flowing recently. Just know
I'm thinking of you, lifting you in prayer, and holding you in
my heart. I empathize with your pain and suffering and
understand the depression and anxiety that result from
everything you've been through. I also know that it seems like
your suffering is compounded daily by many smaller problems,
problems that at any other time would have been manageable
but are now too overwhelming to deal with. Know that you
will get through this, that tomorrow will be a little bit easier,
and the following day a little easier still. Once you stare down
one problem, the next one will be a little more manageable.
You'll find a new normal.

To you who suffer from physical or mental pain/disease,
know that:

He will wipe every tear from their eyes. There will be no
more death or mourning or crying or pain, for the old order of
things has passed away.
Revelation 21:4 ESV

To anyone and everyone in need of encouragement:

I have told you these things, so that in me you may have peace. In this world you will have trouble. But take heart! I have overcome the world.
John 16:33

We are hard pressed on every side, but not crushed; perplexed, but not in despair; persecuted, but not abandoned; struck down, but not destroyed.
2 Corinthians 4:8-9 ESV

The Lord himself goes before you and will be with you; he will never leave you nor forsake you. Do not be afraid; do not be discouraged.
Deuteronomy 31:8 ESV

When Pain Prevents Sleep

"And now my soul is poured out because of my plight;
The days of affliction take hold of me.
My bones are pierced in me at night,
And my gnawing pains take no rest.
Job 30:16-17 NKJV

Some of my friends cannot sleep and cannot rest due to physical pain or illness. I was trying to find bible verses for them that tied in pain and rest, and found these.

Whenever I'm suffering, I always turn to Job. Nothing can compare to what he went through. Because of his pain, he couldn't possibly sleep. (See Job 30:16-17 above).

James tells us what to do when someone is sick:

Is anyone among you sick? Let him call for the elders of the church, and let them pray over him, anointing him with oil in the name of the Lord. And the prayer of faith will save the one who is sick, and the Lord will raise him up. And if he has committed sins, he will be forgiven. Therefore, confess your sins to one another and pray for one another, that you may be healed. The prayer of a righteous person has great power as it is working.
James 5:14-16 ESV

David can rest amid all he's going through because the Lord watches over him and protects him:

I lay down and slept; I woke again, for the Lord sustained me.
Psalm 3:5 ESV

There's a point when, no matter what's keeping us from rest, we become so exhausted that our bodies say "enough," and we get that deep, restorative sleep that we need; even Jesus' human body had to give in to the exhaustion, so much so that He slept through a storm on the sea.

And Jesus said to him, "Foxes have holes, and birds of the air have nests,

but the Son of Man has nowhere to lay his head."
Matthew 8:20 ESV

And behold, there arose a great storm on the sea,

so that the boat was being swamped by the waves; but he was asleep.
Matthew 8:24 ESV

I am praying for you. May God give you rest.

Faith as a Mustard Seed

...if you have faith as a mustard seed, you will say to this mountain,
'Move from here to there,' and it will move;
and nothing will be impossible for you.
Matthew 17:20b

Meditation & Journaling:

Take some time to count your blessings. Write them out and refer to them whenever you're feeling down.

_____

_____

_____

_____

_____

_____

_____

_____

_____

_____

Day 7

Heal Me, Save Me

Heal me, O Lord, and I shall be healed;
Save me, and I shall be saved,
For You are my praise.
Jeremiah 17:14 NKJV

Meditation & Journaling:

How was your week? Take a few minutes to write down your thoughts, what happened, and how you feel now compared with the beginning of the week. Write down any "aha" moments you had.

Who have you asked to pray for you? Who are you praying for?

What other thoughts do you want to write down?

_____

_____

_____

_____

_____

_____

_____

WEEK 2
SUFFERING

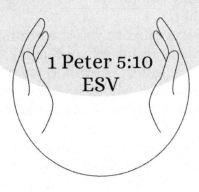

And after you have suffered a little while, the God of all grace, who has called you to his eternal glory in Christ, will himself restore, confirm, strengthen, and establish you.

1 Peter 5:10
ESV

Suffering

More than that, we rejoice in our sufferings,
knowing that suffering produces endurance,
and endurance produces character,
and character produces hope,
and hope does not put us to shame,
because God's love has been poured into our hearts
through the Holy Spirit who has been given to us.
Romans 5:3-5 ESV

It's difficult to think about, but our loving God may have a purpose for our pain.

Has God ever revealed to you something good or positive that's happened as a result of your pain? Maybe you were reconnected with a family member, or you were able to encourage someone else who's suffering. Or, by witnessing your steadfast faith, someone came to accept Jesus as their Lord and Savior.

My first husband developed colon cancer and died three years later. Initially, I asked God, "Why did he die?" but after spending some time praying on it, I discovered the question I should have been asking was, "Why did he live?" I could reflect on the aspects of his life that were a blessing to me and my family and those who knew him. He touched many lives. Because he got colon cancer, a lot of people decided to get colonoscopies who wouldn't have before. Many of them had pre-cancerous polyps removed and lived longer. Each of them then touched many more lives.

While sick, my husband encouraged others with his attitude and perseverance. In the last few months of his life, he was drawn closer to God and spent time in prayer, something he hadn't done for decades.

It's easy to focus on the pain and suffering, but that often leads to depression, bitterness, and hostility. Instead of focusing on the suffering itself, let's see how God uses that suffering for good. We don't live in a vacuum. Our actions and reactions affect numerous people each and every day.

Dear GOD: please help me through this time of pain and suffering. Please help me rejoice in my suffering so that it may produce endurance, character, and hope. Let me never be put to shame, for I know it is Your love that has been poured into my heart. Your sacred gift of the Holy Spirit guides me through the good times and the bad. Lord, I am so very thankful. In Jesus' name, I pray. Amen.

Joseph Suffered

And we know that for those who love God
all things work together for good,
for those who are called according to his purpose.
Romans 8:28 ESV

I don't want to approach this week of prayer with the question: "Why does God allow suffering?" Instead, we're here to look at it from a different viewpoint. We will look at it from the perspective of "Why God allows suffering." I believe the question represents our disapproval of how God handles things, whereas the statement shows our confidence in God's sovereignty.

The best example of this is Joseph. Here was a teenager (17), the youngest of eleven, favored by his father, Jacob. His siblings despised him. After Joseph shared two dreams with them in which they bowed down to him, they couldn't take it anymore. They sold him to some passersby, who sold him into slavery. He ended up in Egypt and eventually found favor with Pharaoh. Through a series of events you'll have to read about on your own (see Genesis 37-48 for the entire event), Joseph saved everyone, including his family, from starvation during a seven-year famine. Did Joseph suffer? Yes. Did God use Joseph's suffering for His plan? Yes, most definitely. If he hadn't been sold into slavery, thousands of people would have died during the famine.

I know this is an extreme example, but it's one where we can see it as a whole, from beginning to end. If we could do that in our own lives, we might better understand God's purpose for our suffering.

Dear GOD: I know deep down that all things work for those who love You. I know that I am called according to Your purpose. But, dear Lord, I am struggling. Some days, the pain is so bad that I can't even get out of bed. I feel helpless and abandoned. Father, I pray that You'll remind me of Your loving presence, especially on my worst days. I praise You, dear Father, for hearing me when no one else does. I lean on Your sovereignty. In Jesus' precious name, I pray. Amen.

Assurance in Suffering

"Neither this man nor his parents sinned,
but that the works of God should be revealed in him.
John 9:3 NKJV

I love that when I'm in the Word, God provides information from it as research for our prayer group. I'm in multiple bible study groups, and each has seemingly overlapped over the past few weeks. Two verses stood out:

Now as Jesus passed by, He saw a man who was blind from birth. And His disciples asked Him, saying, "Rabbi, who sinned, this man or his parents, that he was born blind?"

Jesus answered, "Neither this man nor his parents sinned, but that the works of God should be revealed in him.
John 9:1-3 NKJV

He has not dealt with us according to our sins,

Nor punished us according to our iniquities.
Psalm 103:10 NKJV

Remember these passages whenever life gets you down, and draw hope from them.

When my late husband discovered that his cancer was stage 4, he kept saying that God hated him. God didn't hate him. God used his disease to save other people's lives and draw us closer to Him. I'm sure there were several different ways that God used it for His purposes.

The other part was that since we have free will, our decisions can considerably impact what happens to us. There are consequences for our actions. My husband drank a lot, which predisposed him to colon cancer. For years, he felt like something was wrong but never saw a doctor. Those two decisions led to unfavorable consequences.

However, I draw reassurance in knowing that whatever is going on in my life, God will ultimately use it for good.

Dear GOD: I know that it's nothing I did to bring this pain upon myself. I understand that You have a purpose for me and that my condition may play a part in it, that You may be glorified through it. I will remain patient and trusting, knowing that everything You do is for a purpose and will occur in Your perfect timing. Thank You, dear Lord, for loving me. In Jesus' name, I pray. Amen.

Day 11

Trust in the Lord

For our light affliction,
which is but for a moment,
is working for us a far more exceeding
and eternal weight of glory,
2 Corinthians 4:17 NKJV

A week isn't nearly long enough to illustrate all of the people who suffered greatly throughout the Bible. But I would be remiss if I didn't mention the One who suffered the most: Christ Jesus, the Son of God. Jesus suffered for all of us, bearing the full wrath of God, the wrath that was meant for us. He was falsely accused, spat upon, beaten, and humiliated. He deserved none of it but endured it all.

Paul also suffered much. He was tortured and jailed repeatedly for his faith, as presently happens to people in multiple countries. Yet, he wrote to the Corinthians the above message, calling it their light affliction, reminding them that it is but for a moment and that their suffering in this world is nothing compared to the eternal weight of glory.

No matter what we're going through, it will pass, and we'll come through stronger for having endured. I'm not minimizing our daily sufferings; suffering is suffering. But I want to encourage you to pray and to dig deep into His word for strength and answers. Trust in the Lord, with all your heart (Proverbs 3:5).

Dear GOD: please help me with my affliction. The pain consumes me, and it isn't easy to focus on anything else. Please help me overcome this. Please show me the way. In Jesus' precious name, I pray. Amen.

Peace in Christ

These things I have spoken to you,
that in Me you may have peace.
In the world you will have tribulation;
but be of good cheer, I have overcome the world."
John 16:33 NKJV

I find a lot of comfort in this verse. We can find peace in Christ. In this world, this life, things are difficult because sin entered the world long ago. But I'm learning to hand everything in this life over to Jesus. There are things I can't handle, things I can't do anything about, but Jesus can. He overcame this world. He overcame death. He sits at the right hand of God. Nothing is impossible for Him, and we have His Spirit inside each of us to guide the way.

Rest in Him and find your peace.

Dear GOD: I am so thankful for what You've done for me. I'm grateful for the blessings. Most of all, I am thankful for the peace and hope You give me each and every day. Please use me, dear Lord, to be Your image-bearer. In Jesus' name, I pray. Amen.

Testing of Your Faith

Count it all joy, my brothers and sisters,
when you meet trials of various kinds,
for you know that the testing of your faith
produces steadfastness.
And let steadfastness have its full effect,
that you may be perfect and complete,
lacking in nothing.
James 1:2-4 ESV

Meditation & Journaling:

Write a prayer. What do you want to say to God about your own suffering? What do you want to ask Him or tell Him?

_____

_____

_____

_____

_____

_____

_____

God Will Restore You

And after you have suffered a little while,
the God of all grace,
who has called you to his eternal glory in Christ,
will himself restore, confirm, strengthen, and
establish you.
1 Peter 5:10 ESV

Meditation & Journaling:

How was your week? Take a few minutes to write down your thoughts, what happened, and how you feel now compared with the beginning of the week. Write down any "aha" moments you had.

Has your attitude toward your suffering changed? Have you thought of any occurrences where God used your pain to help others?

_____

_____

_____

_____

_____

_____

PEACE

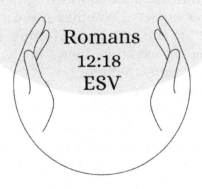

If possible, so far as it depends on you, live peaceably with all.

Romans
12:18
ESV

Cast Off Your Burdens

Cast your burden on the Lord,
And He shall sustain you;
He shall never permit the righteous to be shaken.
Psalm 55:22 NKJV

At the height of my anxiety, I met a woman online who had just as much going on as I did, if not more. Every day, she said she was okay because she was giving it up to the Lord. She said she didn't have to worry about it because she cast that burden on God, and He was comforting her and working in her life, easing her anxiety. Whether she was actually able to distance herself from the pain and suffering, I don't know, but I started following her example. I gave my worries to God and asked Him to take care of them for me. It took a lot of practice, but it helped tremendously.

Jesus bore the ultimate burden by dying on the cross to pay our debt. We know a love so pure that it can wipe away our sins and give us eternal life. We can rest in this amazing love, grace, and mercy. Others will see the peace within us and want what we have, which will bring glory to our Lord. So, no matter what's going on in your life, try to give it all to God! In doing so, you'll glorify Him.

Dear GOD, I give You this burden which I carry. I can no longer bear it alone. The pain is intense and wears on my physical, emotional, and spiritual well-being. I want the peace that comes from trusting in You. Please help me, Lord. In Jesus' name, I pray. Amen.

Lift Up My Eyes to the Hills

I lift up my eyes to the hills.
From where does my help come?
My help comes from the Lord,
who made heaven and earth.
He will not let your foot be moved;
he who keeps you will not slumber.
Psalm 121:1-3 ESV

My experience has been that when I give my problems to the Lord, my load seems lessened, and my problems or worries seem smaller, more manageable. I'm able to think clearly.

Someone posted this quote yesterday, and it brought things into perspective for me:

"Today is the tomorrow you worried about yesterday." ~ Dale Carnegie

I tried to remember all the things I've worried about this week, and did any of them happen? Did my worries do anyone any good? The answer to both questions is "no."

Then, I looked at what I've prayed for this week, and were any of them answered? Did my prayers do anyone any good? The answer to both questions is "yes."

God is here for us. We need Him. We can't go this alone. Let's look to Him when we feel helpless. Lean on Him.

Dear GOD: I pray that I remember to "lift up my eyes to the hills" because that is where You reside, and where You are is where my help comes from. I praise You for watching over me and protecting me. In Jesus' name, I pray. Amen.

Perfect Peace

You will keep him in perfect peace,
Whose mind is stayed on You,
Because he trusts in You.
Trust in the Lord forever,
For in YAH, the Lord, is everlasting strength.*
Isaiah 26:3-4 NKJV
*"everlasting strength" means "Rock of Ages."

Have you ever experienced "perfect peace?" I have during specific points of my life. Every experience of perfect peace followed a time of getting closer to God, listening to Him, and understanding His will for what He wants me to do.

How often do you set aside time to listen? I know many excellent and faithful "pray-ers," but seemingly, few realize they must sit still and listen for a response.

When we pray, we engage in a conversation with our Heavenly Father, but if we don't listen for His response, then we're simply engaging in a monologue. Trust in Him to answer. It may not be an immediate response, but give Him that space anyway. Trust in Him. He will provide perfect peace. He is our Rock of Ages.

Dear GOD: please grant peace and comfort during periods of pain, especially when our suffering is at its worst. Please heal our loved ones and ourselves. The constant, nagging, unrelenting pain is so overwhelming. Please help us. Please give us that perfect peace that can only be achieved through trust in You. In Jesus' name, we pray. Amen.

Day 18

Live Peaceably

If possible, so far as it depends on you, live peaceably with all.
Romans 12:18 ESV

We need to take off the glasses that make us label everyone. We who suffer from chronic pain are often labeled by those who don't even try to understand us. Some consider us to be lazy, whiners, and weak. People always have a quick fix for us, "If you would exercise, lose weight, eat healthier, try this or that supplement, or _____ (fill in the blank), you'd feel a lot better." Trust me, if there were an easy fix, I would have done it by now.

Some doctors look at our charts instead of at us and determine that, since we're taking antidepressants and/or anti-anxiety medicine, the pain is all in our heads. They prescribe a 30-minute walk five days a week as if that's the cure for everything.

What hurts more than our physical pain and the heartless blow-off from supposed "specialists," is the lack of empathy from our loved ones. Not that we're trying to get sympathy, just an acknowledgment of our very real condition. We may need help with daily activities or just a warm hug.

I chose this Bible verse because we must forgive those who hurt us. If we didn't, we would, undoubtedly, be utterly alone. I've clung to grudges, even hatred, in my lifetime, and it does me more damage than it does the other person. We each carry our own cross and trust in the Lord to see us through the obstacles of this earthly existence.

Dear GOD: please grant us the ability to live peaceably with all. Please reveal our pain to our loved ones so they can support us and love on us and us on them. In Jesus' name, we pray. Amen.

Lean on Jesus

Now may the Lord of peace himself
give you peace at all times in every way.
The Lord be with you all.
2 Thessalonians 3:16 ESV

No matter what you're going through, lean on the Lord for comfort, healing, and strength. Praise Him for His unwavering love. Ask Him the hard questions and listen for an answer.

Shortly after I was diagnosed with breast cancer and was facing many months of radiation and chemotherapy, I cried out to the Lord and asked, "What good am I to You now? How can I serve You like this?"

A few minutes later, the phone rang. It was a national charity that I had sent a small amount of money to recently. The person said she was calling to thank me for my donation. They never did that before, and they have never done it since. It was God providing an answer to my prayer. My husband and I were big on supporting various Christian charities, and the Lord reminded me that this was a way to serve.

I didn't realize this until years later, but what I went through during my cancer journey supplied me with dozens of testimonies that I can share with those who are suffering. So, yes, God can use all things for His purposes. We don't always get to know the why, but we can trust in Him. He's got us.

Dear GOD: I'm in constant pain. How is this according to Your will? How is this life serving You, bringing glory to You? Father, I wish to let go of my pain. I hand it over to You. I also give You my life that You will use me to help others. Please provide me with comfort, healing, and strength through this trial. In Jesus' name, I pray. Amen.

Peace of Christ

And let the peace of Christ rule in your hearts,
to which indeed you were called in one body.
And be thankful.
Colossians 3:15 ESV

Meditation & Journaling:

Meditate on this verse. How can you find the peace of Christ? Ask God to grant you Christ's peace. Praise Him and thank Him when He gives this to you. Write down your question for God and His response.

_____

_____

_____

_____

_____

_____

_____

_____

_____

_____

In Peace

There are many who say, "Who will show us some good?
Lift up the light of your face upon us, O Lord!"
You have put more joy in my heart
than they have when their grain and wine abound.
In peace I will both lie down and sleep;
for you alone, O Lord, make me dwell in safety.
Psalm 4:6-8 ESV

Meditation & Journaling:

How was your week? Take a few minutes to write down your thoughts, what happened, and how you feel now compared with the beginning of the week. Write down any "aha" moments you had.

Can you find safety in the Lord? How?

_____

_____

_____

_____

_____

_____

_____

WEEK 4
HOPE

Now hope does not disappoint, because the love of God has been poured out in our hearts by the Holy Spirit who was given to us.

Romans 5:5
NKJV

God of Hope

May the God of hope fill you with all joy and
peace in believing, so that by the power
of the Holy Spirit you may abound in hope.
Romans 15:13 ESV

Sometimes, with chronic conditions, we go through the grief stages. It's challenging to handle that our lives are forever changed and to face the possibility that we may no longer do the things we once enjoyed and looked forward to. We are grieving for our pre-illness life.

The stages are denial, anger, bargaining, depression, and acceptance. We may go through all of the stages or just a few. We may go through them in order or not. No matter what stage you may find yourself in, know that you can find peace and hope in God.

Denial - Ask God to help you through this stage. It's probably the hardest one to pray through because we don't recognize that there's a problem. It's an excellent time to research what the doctor has told you and to seek help from others who are going through what you are. I joined 3 Facebook groups and felt heard and supported when I needed it the most.

Anger - It's natural to lash out at what hurts us or what we don't understand. Expending energy this way doesn't help anyone (not that it can be helped). Ask God for direction.

Bargaining - God doesn't barter, but He does comfort us when we seek Him.

Depression - This may be the most prevalent stage of all. I've found myself stuck in this loop numerous times. I try to turn my mood around by praying more and diving into Scripture. I have conversations with God. Additionally, I (try to) turn my focus away from my pain and toward something else, such as my numerous blessings.

Acceptance - if you find yourself in this stage, hallelujah! Now, you're ready to face this illness head-on with the help of your Heavenly Father. Praise Him!

Dear GOD: we turn to You through any and all stages. You are our Rock and our Fortress, as well as our Redeemer. Our hope is in You alone. Please fill us with "all joy and peace in believing, so that by the power of the Holy Spirit [we] may abound in hope." In Jesus' name, we pray. Amen.

Be True

Jesus wept.
John 11:35 NKJV

It is the shortest verse in the Bible and, in my opinion, the most powerful. Lazarus' mourners so moved Jesus that He also cried.

I imagine Jesus feels all our pains and sorrows, crying when we cry, rejoicing when we rejoice, yet we often hide our negative emotions from the world. We may think our genuine emotions make us appear weak; perhaps we're too full of pride to let others share in our sorrows and pain. We don't want others to know that we're depressed and hurting. We would rather suffer alone. It's so senseless and even hypocritical. I do it, too. When someone asks me how I am or feel, I'll answer "fine" or even "good" when I'm a fragile mess beneath that cheery facade.

We may not want to create an awkward situation by saying we're in pain. Or, maybe we don't want to talk about it, but we're also denying that friend the opportunity to help or comfort us.

I overheard a waitress training someone. She said, "If you're having a bad day, just put on a big smile, and soon you'll feel better." That could be good advice, and it could help, but really, you're putting on a fragile veil that you hope others won't look past so that you can suffer alone.

I get it. I do this, too. There's a fine line between sharing and burdening sometimes, but if you're talking to a family member or faithful friend, that barrier can be broken repeatedly and repaired each time.

I'm a bundle of emotions right now. I'm depressed, frustrated, and exhausted, yet day after day, I let on that I'm strong, all better, and life is back to normal. I don't want other people to feel awkward, I don't want to be "that" person who does nothing but complain, and I don't want to bring them down with me.

I've been very emotional. I've wept.

Dear GOD: I pray that You help me through the low periods when my pain affects my mood and relationships. I know You understand and are probably weeping right along with me. It is a blessing to bring all of this to You, day after day, without worries, because I know You care. In Jesus' name, I pray. Amen.

All We Can Do is Pray

And whatever you ask in My name, that I will do,
that the
Father may be glorified in the Son.
John 14:13 NKJV

If you abide in Me, and My words abide in you, you
will ask what you desire, and it shall be done for you.
John 15:7 NKJV

There is a woman who worries to the point of excess. Not only
does she worry about family and friends, but also about things
that have nothing to do with her. She builds up these 'what if'
scenarios in her mind about things that could go wrong, some
of which are so creative and outlandish that it scares me.

I've tried to convince her that she suffers from anxiety,
but she doesn't believe me and, therefore, won't do anything
about it. The physical results of this are high blood pressure
and a stroke. So then I worry. It's a vicious cycle, isn't it?
Worry begets worry. Anxiety begets anxiety. All of it takes a
toll on us.

As I was preparing to write this, I realized it all comes
down to control. I can't do anything about the actions and
decisions of others, so I'm going to worry about them. At least
in that way, I'm *doing* something. It fills two needs within us:

- to be in charge
- to help others

How often have you said or heard others say, "All we can do is pray?" All we can do--as in, we can't do anything. Oh well. At least praying makes us feel like we're doing something. That is just so wrong! Praying should be our **first** defense! It's THE prize, not the consolation prize!

Jesus prayed all the time. Would He do that if it were just an exercise in futility? Do you think Jesus prayed because He didn't feel He could do something more substantial? No! Of course not! He did it because it was an essential course of action, and He knew His Father in Heaven heard His prayers.

Our prayers can make a difference in the lives of others. So, whenever you feel helpless or emboldened (in other words, always), pray to our Father, who loves us.

Dear GOD: I know that You hear my prayers. I consider it an honor to be called a child of God, one who can converse with the one, true, living God, Creator of the universe. I hope I always have the desire to talk to You each and every day. I pray that our relationship grows stronger and that You reveal more of Yourself, Your perfect characteristics. Father, I praise You, and I love You. In Jesus' name, I pray. Amen.

Where is Your Hope?

For in this hope we were saved. Now hope that is seen is not hope.
For who hopes for what he sees? But if we hope for what we do
not see, we wait for it with patience.
Romans 8:24-25 ESV

The Pastor ended a recent sermon with two questions for us:
- Where's your hope?
- Do friends and family know where your hope is?

I know the correct answer is, "My hope is in Jesus," but honestly, I sometimes struggle with it.

To me, "hope" means something we're uncertain of. I "hope" it won't rain today. I "hope" my friend will heal. Why isn't it "my faith is in Jesus," instead of my hope? I don't know. I'm just asking.

I do know that all of Scripture is God-breathed and that every word has a purpose, so I don't mean to question it in that respect. When I strayed from God, I felt no hope in any situation. That may be the answer. Having faith gives us the hope to persevere throughout this life and guide us into the next.

Dear GOD: we are so grateful for Jesus sacrificing His life for our sins. We are in awe of this free gift You offer us. Because of Your love, we have hope in the life to come. We are thankful that You have given us this hope to help us through this life so we can keep our eyes on the prize to the next life. Father, we pray for those who do not yet have this hope. Many of us remember when we didn't have it and what it felt like. We pray that You will use us to share that hope with everyone we meet. In Jesus' name, we pray. Amen.

Day 26

Hope Does Not Disappoint

Now hope does not disappoint, because the love of God
has been poured out in our hearts by the Holy Spirit
who was given to us.
Romans 5:5 NKJV

I only realized how much Paul wrote about hope in Christ
when I began this week's study. He was quite the encourager.
He was also candid and stern when necessary.
  - Through Paul's letters, God reveals the truths of the New
  Covenant and demonstrates how to be a true Christ-
  follower by showing Paul's heart and character. He has a
  deep love and commitment to other followers.
  - He trusts God entirely for all of his needs.
  - He shares the gospel with everyone he meets.
  - He speaks the truth without sugar-coating it.
  - Everything he does and says is for the glory of God.
  Today's Bible verse shows us just how much God loves us.
He is constantly "pouring out" His love. I feel disgraced that
I'm not pouring out my love for Abba every moment of every
day.

Dear GOD: words cannot express how much I love You. Please
guide me and order my steps so that I may be more Christlike
and that I may share my passion for You as Paul did. Lord, I

praise You and thank You for Your love and grace. In Jesus' precious name, I pray. Amen.

In a Valley

Every valley shall be exalted
And every mountain and hill brought low;
The crooked places shall be made straight
And the rough places smooth;
Isaiah 40:4 NKJV

When I was going through chemo and radiation, there were days when I was praising God that I was alive, and then there were days when I was crying at the prospect of dying. It was an extremely emotional time made even more difficult by the fact that I had just lost a husband to cancer two years before.

One of the things that got me through was the outpouring of love and support from people worldwide. I had online friends from several countries, and many kept in touch by email, I.M., or social media and let me know that they were praying for me.

What made my day every once in a while was when I would receive a card in the mail. It was just so wonderful to know that someone took the time to buy a card and write a note on it. It never failed to cheer me up.

Now, when I'm down, a wonderful pick-me-up is buying a card or small something for someone I know is sick or hurting. It's my opinion that when I'm depressed, it helps immensely to turn my focus onto others AND to count my blessings.

If you're trapped in a valley or know someone who is, think about sending them a card today, and you may lift both yourself and the card recipient to the mountaintops.

Dear GOD: I lift up the valleys to You and praise You even when the mountains are brought low. May the crooked places be made straight and the rough places be made smooth. May everything be done according to Your perfect plan. You are my Rock and my Redeemer. All that I am is because of You. In Jesus' name, I pray. Amen.

Meditation & Journaling:

Once again, count your blessings. Write them out and look at them when you're feeling low. What can you do to lift yourself up? Have you discussed any problems with God yet? Give it a try. It always helps me.

_____

_____

_____

_____

_____

_____

_____

_____

_____

_____

_____

_____

Pain

Therefore let those who suffer
according to God's will
entrust their souls to a faithful Creator
while doing good.
1 Peter 4:19 ESV

(Note: This post was written several years before I developed Chronic Fatigue Syndrome and Fibromyalgia. I didn't understand what it was like to be in constant pain or to have any chronic issues, so please take what's written here with a grain of salt.)

I am a bit of a baby when I'm in pain for any length of time. I have arthritis and allergy-related headaches, but other than that, I have no pain. So, when I meet someone who is in constant pain and deals with it daily AND still maintains her faith and sunny disposition, I have to look at that person and believe that God is using her to glorify Him.

We are made in His image, and anything we do to show how He is working in our lives, whether it's our disposition, loving-kindness, or how we handle difficult situations, all of it reflects on God. People look at us and want what we have.

They want the peace, comfort, and love they see in us. We can inspire others through our suffering, which glorifies God.

Those who suffer from physical pain who don't know Jesus may have a more difficult time dealing with their pain. I imagine that they do.

When I was going through chemo and radiation therapy, I smiled through it all and tried to help others who were having a more difficult time of it. I had lapses where I felt like I was going to die and mourned what I was going through, but they were temporary breakdowns, and hopefully, others saw in me how God was working through me.

I sincerely hope this doesn't come across as sounding like those in pain need to suffer in silence because you don't. You should get angry when you feel angry, work through the doubt when you feel low, and ask God, "why me?" when questioning His path for you. But, when you're ready to bounce back from those low points, feel His love and support and know He has a reason for everything and everything is part of His plan.

Meditation & Journaling:

Write a prayer to your loving Father. Tell Him how you're feeling. Ask Him the hard questions, and then listen for His answers.

_____

_____

_____

_____

_____

_____

_____

_____

Upcoming Books

from Dear God Ltd.

I sincerely hope this devotional has been a blessing to you. To follow along with my daily posts, please join my Facebook Group, <u>Pray in the Stillness</u>, and/or follow me on <u>Patreon</u>. The free account will get regular updates for new books, products, and accessories to enhance the inspiration from *Dear God: I'm in Pain.*

Coming in early 2024, an anthology: *Letters from the Fold: Seeing God in a Season of Pain.* This book is a collection of inspirational stories from brothers and sisters in Christ who suffer from chronic pain. They share how they've seen God work through the pain and how it's brought them closer to Him.

Follow my <u>Amazon Author Page</u> so you don't miss the release of this encouraging book.

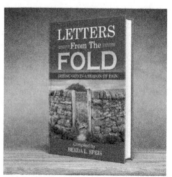

All my links can be found at <u>linktr.ee/beedaspeis</u>

There are two companion books for *Dear God: I'm in Pain*: a pain tracker, and a journal with encouraging Bible verses, prayers, and inspirational quotes. I'm including sample pages for you to try out.

PAIN 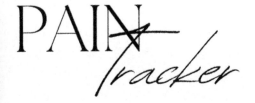 Tracker

PAIN LEVEL TODAY:

| PAIN, WHAT PAIN? | I CAN DO STUFF | TWINGES OF PAIN | NOT QUITE RIGHT | MANAGE -ABLE? |

| NOT GOOD NOT BAD | OTC MEDS | COUCH DAY | AS BAD AS IT GETS | TAKE ME TO THE ER |

SLEEP: _____

Last night I slept From _____ To _____

Naps _____

EXERCISE:

Number of steps _____

Other exercise: _____

Number of minutes: _____

WATER:

💧 💧 💧 💧 💧 💧 💧 💧
1   2   3   4   5   6   7   8   (Glass)

WEATHER:

High/Low: _____

Type of weather: _____

Other conditions: _____

MENTAL HEALTH:

Circle all that apply:

sad   happy   excited   angry

bored   blah   joyful   lost

lonely   depressed   anxious   resentful

Something else: _____

_____

POSSIBLE TRIGGERS:

_____

_____

TODAY I TRIED:

(e.g. Something new to help my pain & mood: supplements, started a new medicine, walked, talked to a friend, dietary changes, etc.)

_____

_____

_____

_____

_____

_____

_____

_____

FOOD:

Breakfast:

_____

_____

Lunch:

_____

_____

Dinner:

_____

_____

Snacks:

_____

_____

CHANGES IN MY ROUTINE TODAY:

_____

_____

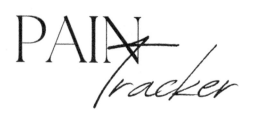

PAIN ~~Tracker~~

DATE: __ / __ / __

● ● ● ● ● ● ●
S M T W T F S

WHAT WENT WELL TODAY?

_____
_____
_____
_____
_____
_____
_____
_____
_____
_____
_____
_____
_____
_____

WHAT DIDN'T GO WELL?

_____
_____
_____
_____
_____
_____
_____
_____
_____
_____
_____
_____
_____
_____
_____
_____
_____

WHAT CAN I DO DIFFERENTLY?

_____
_____
_____
_____

GOALS FOR TOMORROW:

_____
_____
_____
_____
_____

I can do all things through Christ who strengthens me. Philippians 4:13 NKJV

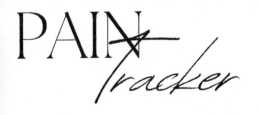

DATE: /   /

● ● ● ● ● ● ●
S   M   T   W   T   F   S

THOUGHTS/IDEAS

Dear God:

Therefore let those who suffer
according to God's will
entrust their souls to a
faithful Creator
while doing good.

1 Peter 4:19 ESV

Father, I lift up the valleys to You and praise You even when the mountains are brought low. May the crooked places be made straight and the rough places be made smooth. May everything be done according to Your perfect plan. You are my Rock and my Redeemer. All that I am is because of You. In Jesus' name, I pray. Amen.

Dear God: I'm in pain.

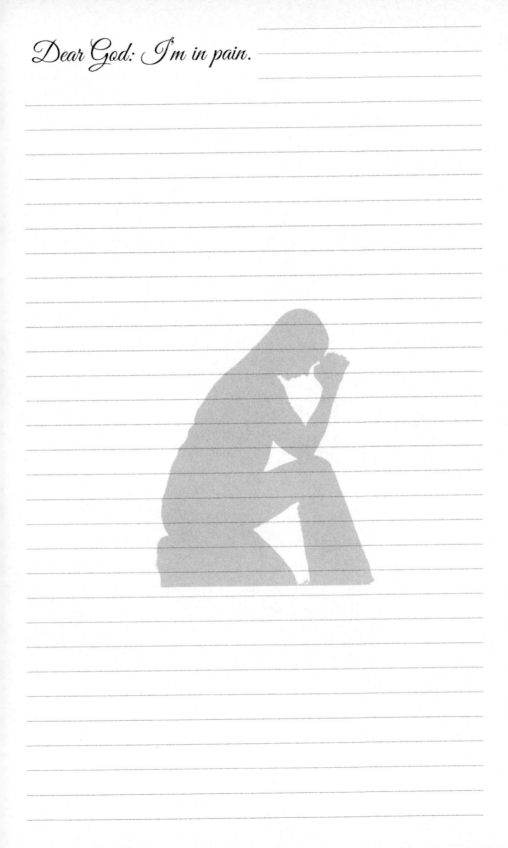

"God whispers to us in our pleasures, speaks in our conscience, but shouts in our pains: it is His megaphone to rouse a deaf world." ~ C.S. Lewisl

If you abide in Me, and My words abide in you, you will ask what you desire, and it shall be done for you.

John 15:7 NKJV

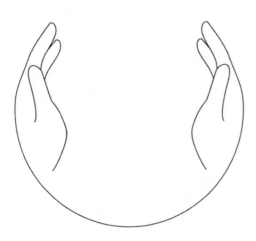

Printed in Great Britain
by Amazon

38524433R00046